The Most Famous DIAMONDS in the World

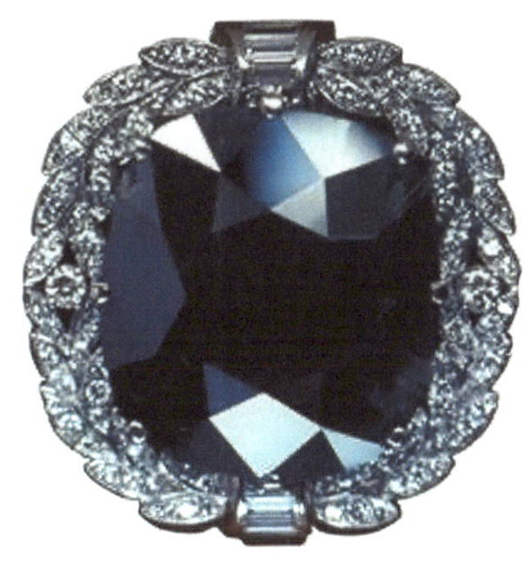

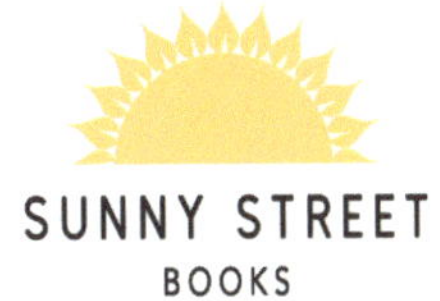

SUNNY STREET
BOOKS

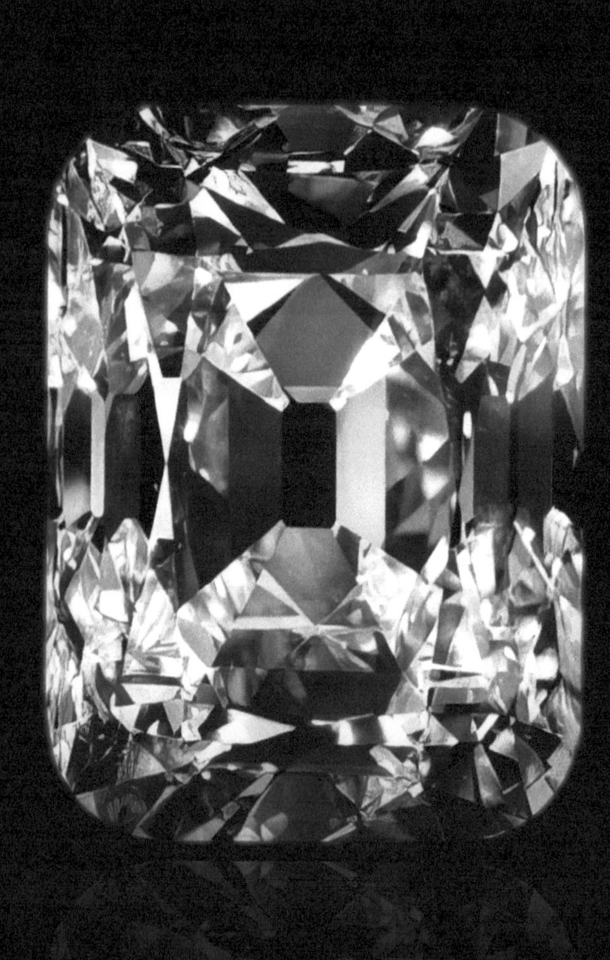

THE BEAU SANCY

Description

Carats: 34.98 carats

Cut: Modified pear, double rose cut

Color: Faint brown

Origin

Discovered in India in the
16th century

Value

$9.7 million

Residence

Undisclosed

THE BLACK ORLOV

Description

Carats: 67.49 carats

Cut: Cushion cut

Color: Black

Origin

Discovered in India in the
19th century

Value

$360,000

Residence

Undisclosed

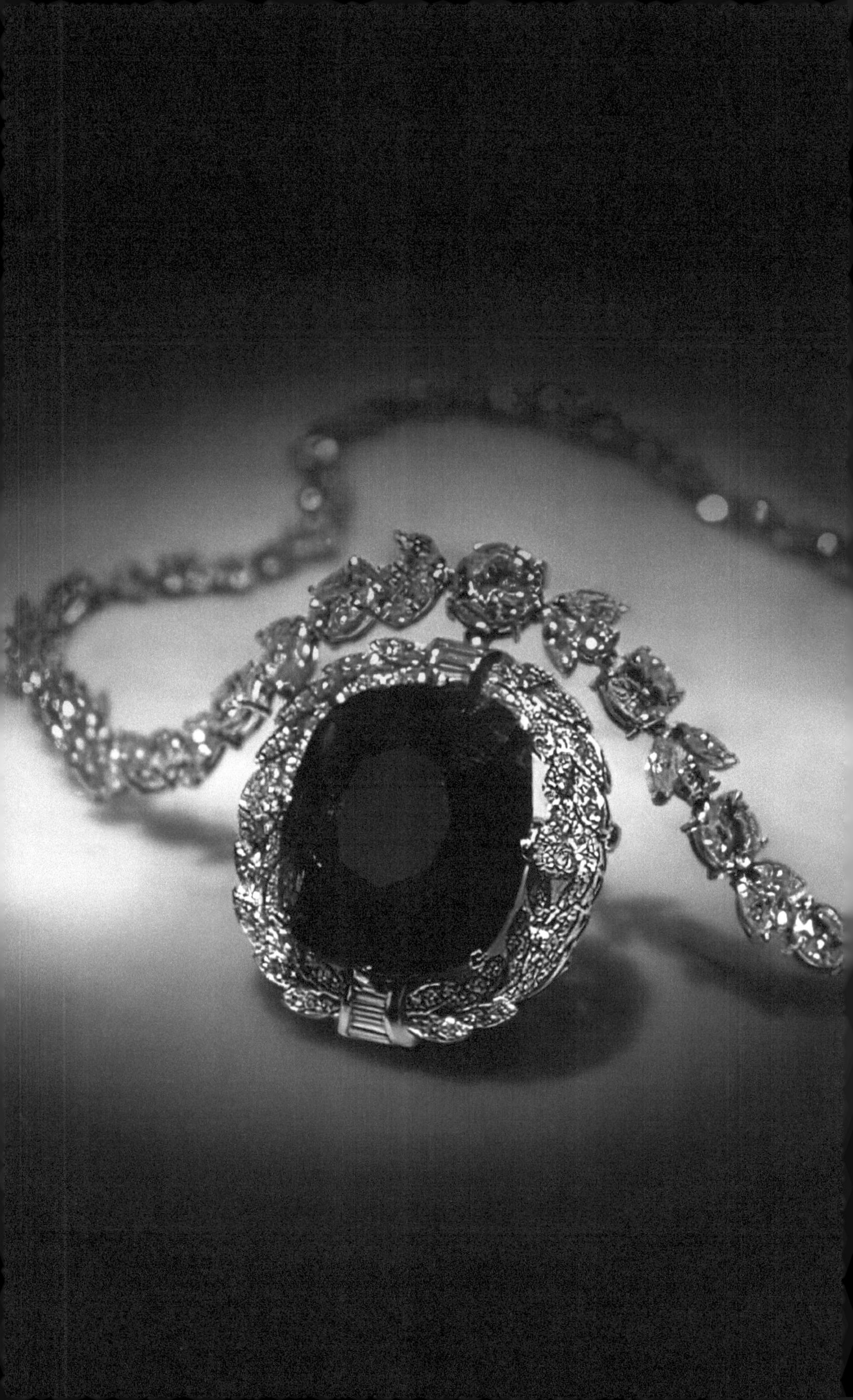

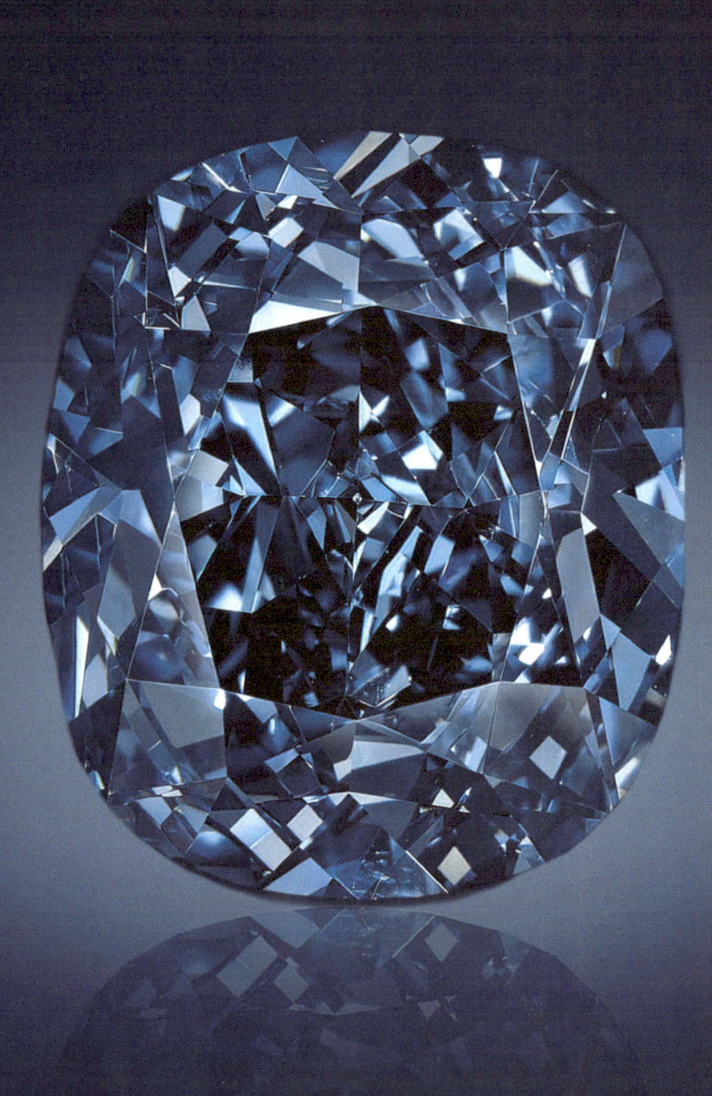

Description

Carats: 12.03 carats

Cut: Cushion cut

Color: Fancy vivid blue

Clarity: Flawless

Origin

Discovered in South Africa

in 2014

Value

$48.4 million

Residence

Owned by Hong Kong billionaire,

Joseph Lau Luen-hung

THE CENTENARY DIAMOND

Description

Carats: 273.85 carats

Cut: Modified heart-shaped brilliant cut

Color: Colorless

Clarity: Flawless

Origin

Discovered in South Africa

in 1986

Value

$100 million

Residence

Undisclosed

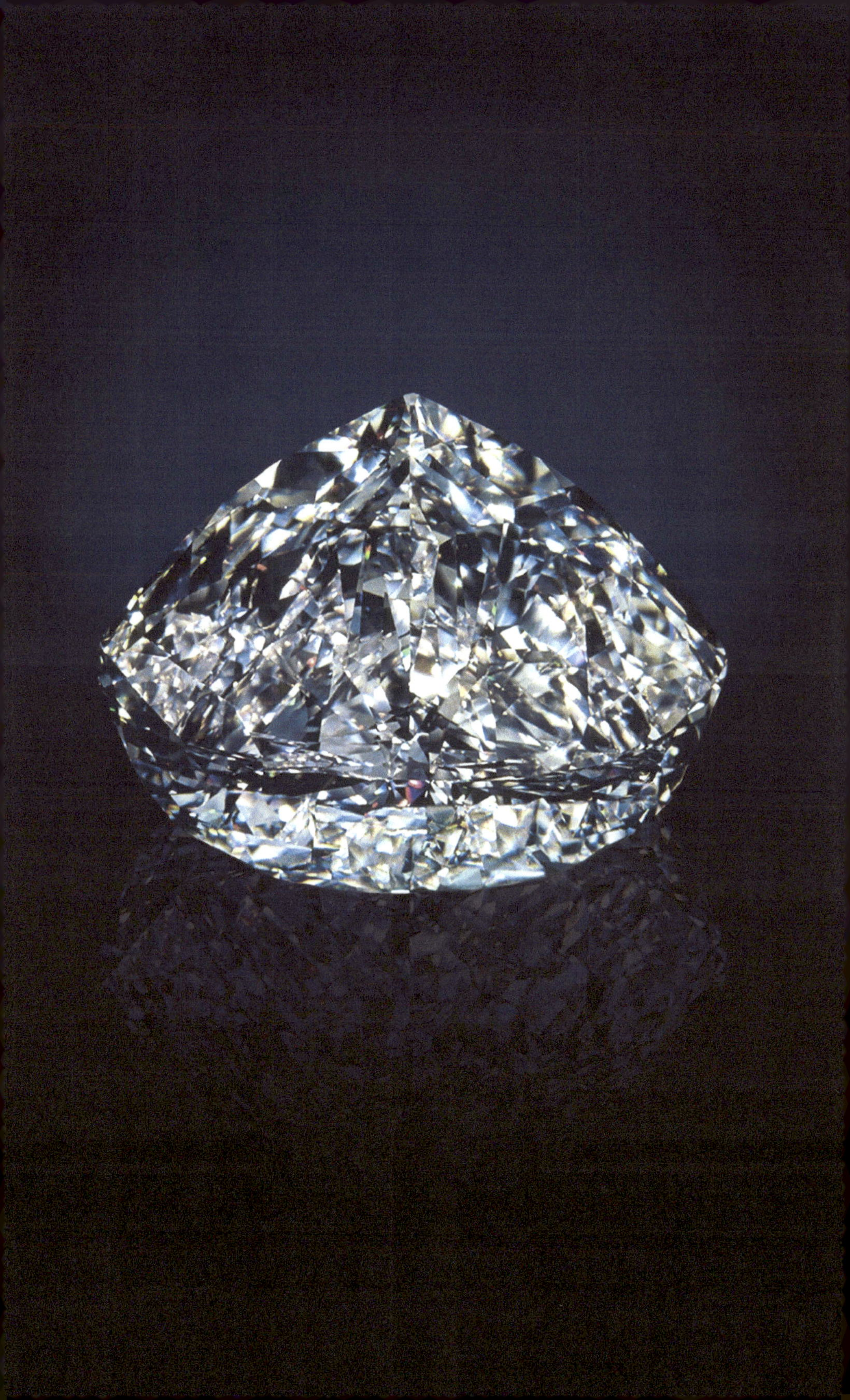

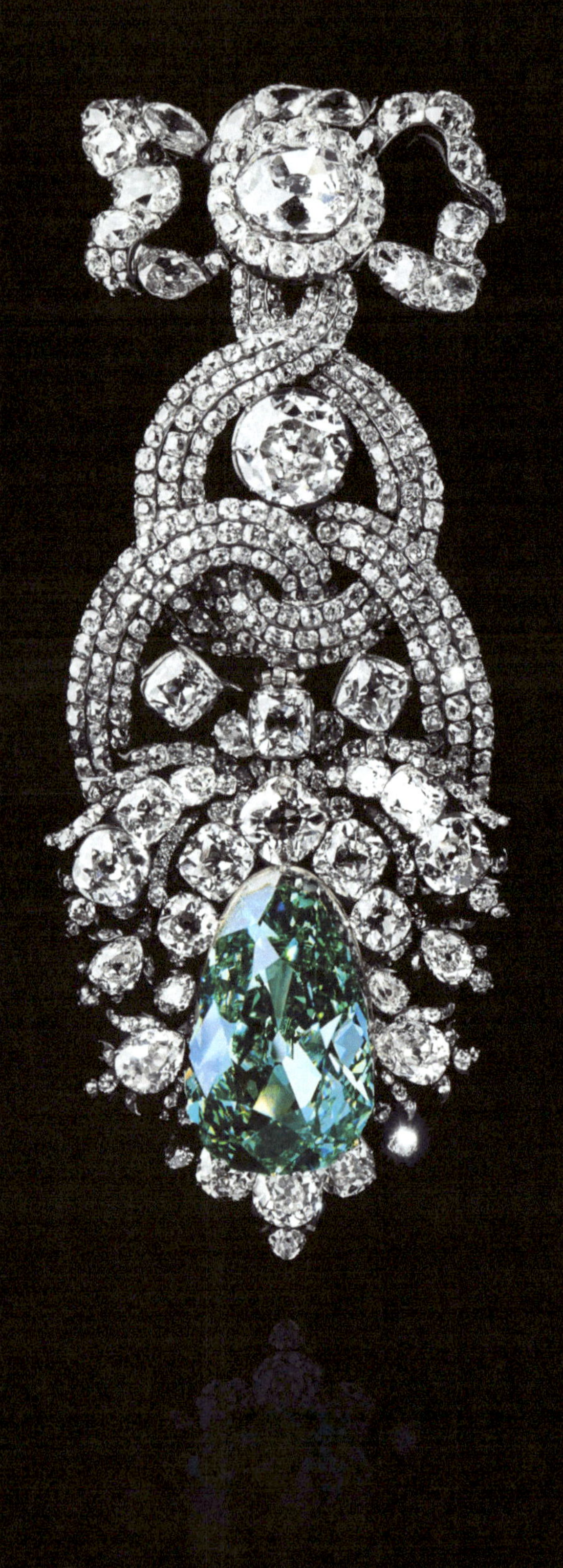

The Dresden Green

Description

Carats: 40.70 carats

Cut: Modified pear-shaped brilliant cut

Color: Fancy medium green

Clarity: Very, very slight inclusions

Origin

Discovered in India in the
18th century

Value

Undetermined

Residence

Albertinium Museum
Dresden, Germany

THE GREAT STAR OF AFRICA

Description

Carats: 530.2 carats

Cut: Pear-shaped cut

Color: Colorless

Origin

Discovered in South Africa

in 1905

Value

Estimated at $400 million

Residence

The Sovereign's Sceptre

of the British Crown Jewels

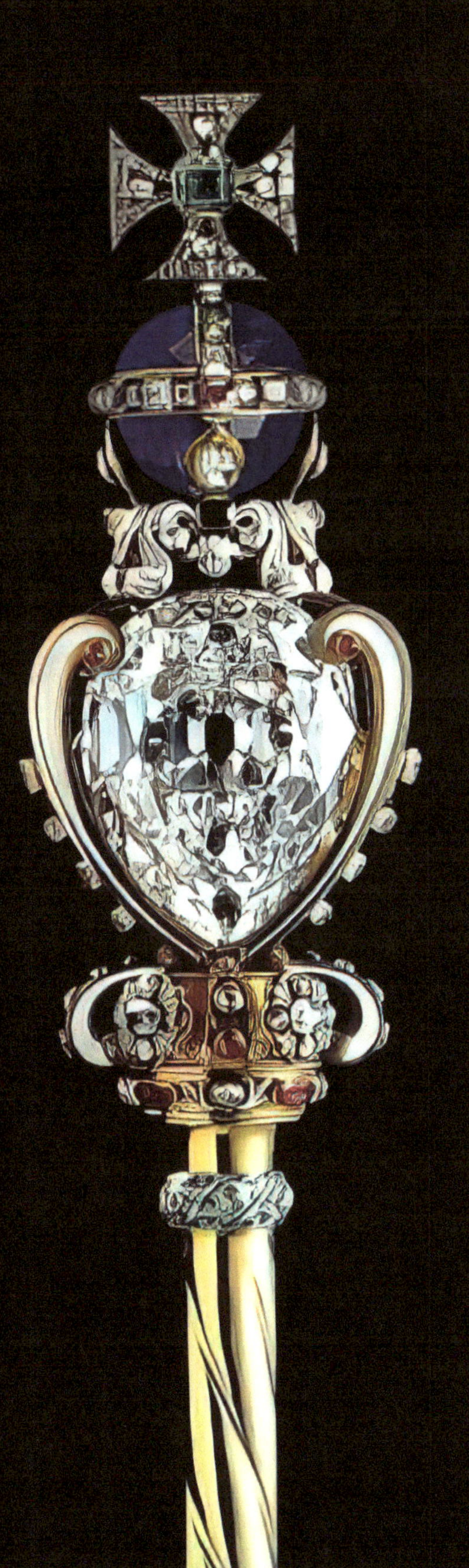

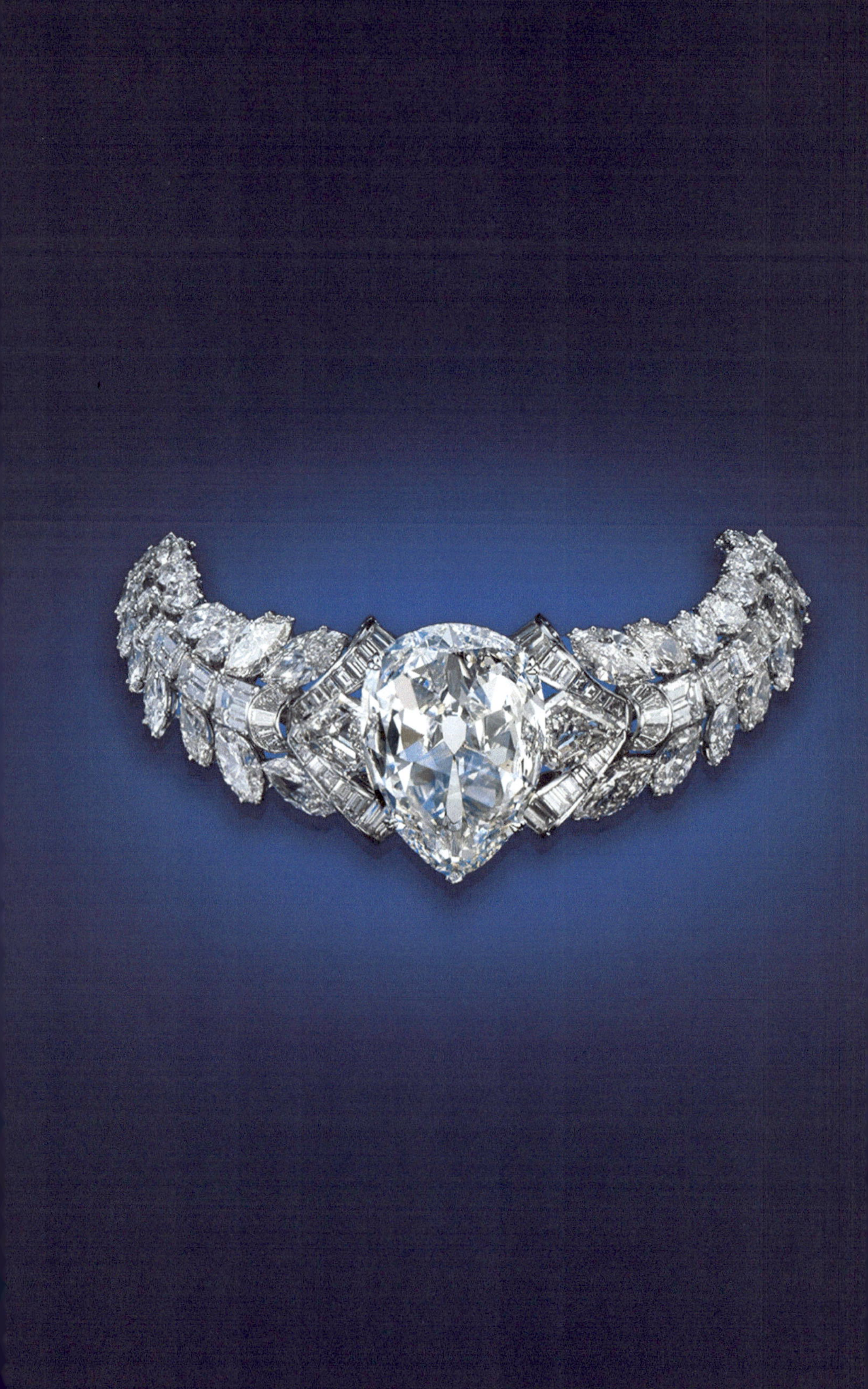

Description

Carats: 69.68 carats

Cut: Pear-shaped cut

Color: Near colorless

Clarity: Slight inclusions

Origin

Discovered in South Africa
in 1893

Value

$2.6 million

Residence

Owned by Robert Mouawad, who set it
in a bracelet as the center stone

Description

Carats: 545.67 carats

Cut: Fire rose cushion cut

Color: Fancy yellow brown

Clarity: Flawless

Origin

Discovered in South Africa
in 1985

Value

Estimated between $4 and $12 million

Residence

Displayed at the Royal Museum
in Bangkok as part of the
Indian Crown Jewels

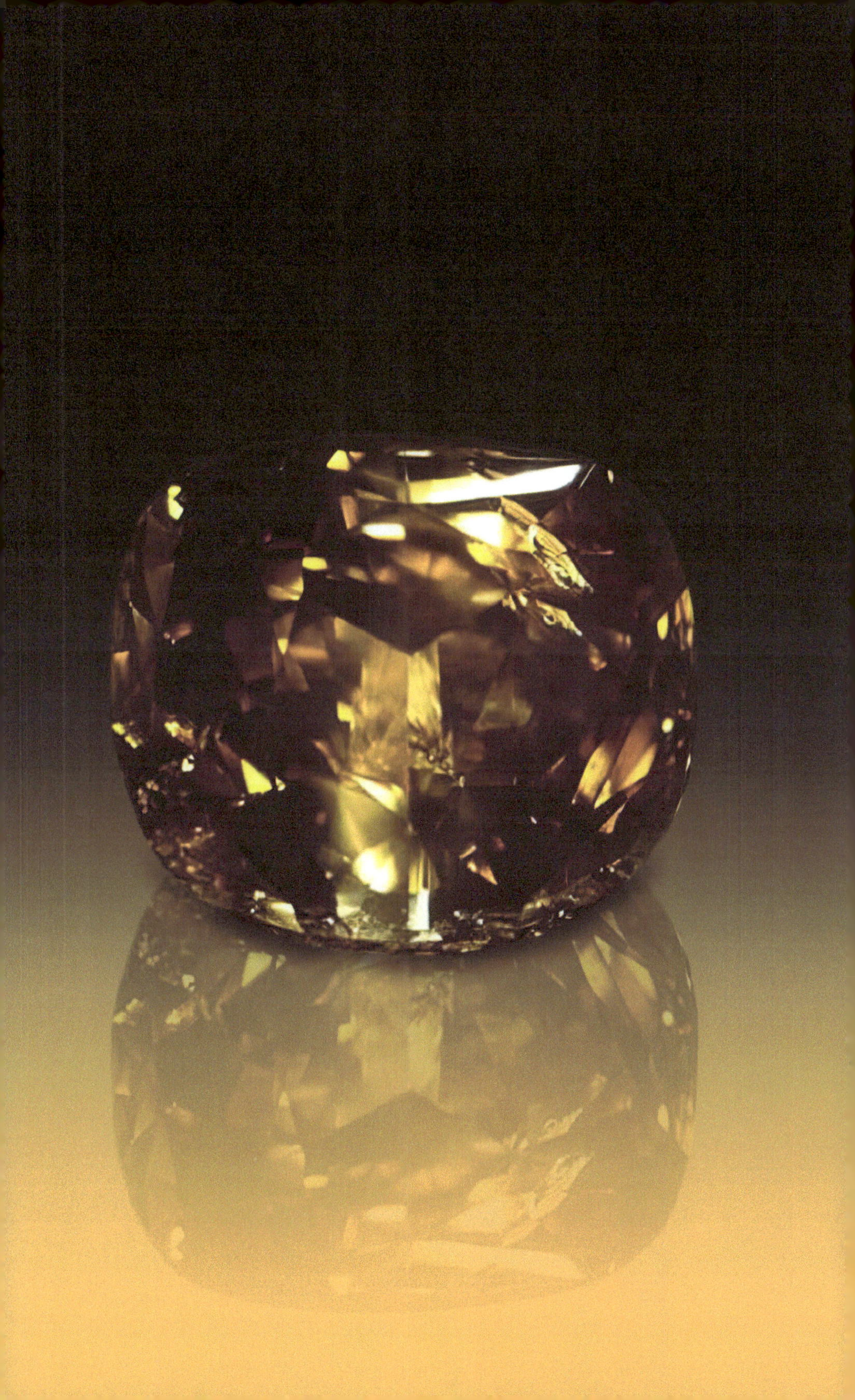

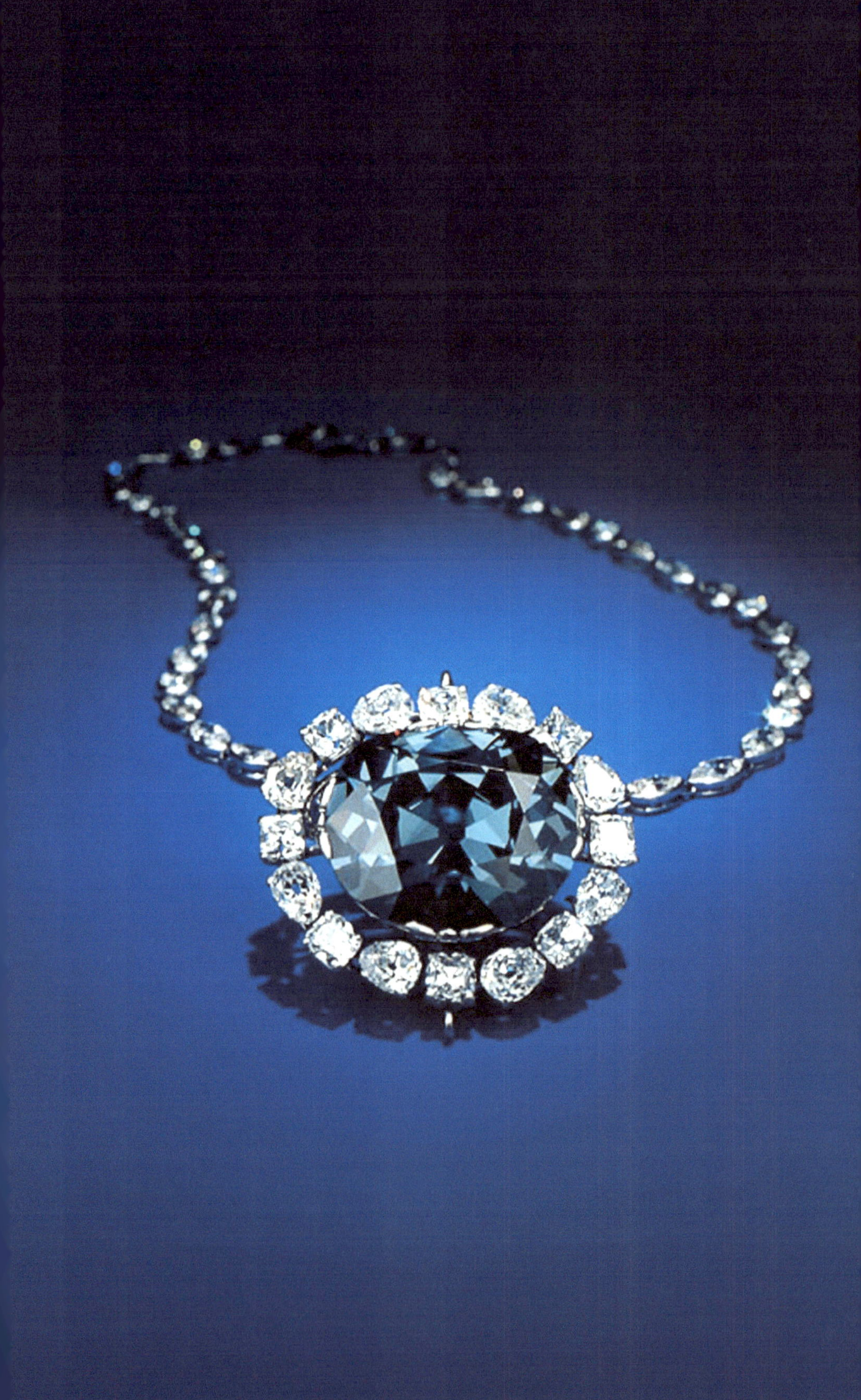

THE HOPE DIAMOND

Description

Carats: 45.52 carats

Cut: Cushion antique brilliant

Color: Fancy deep grayish blue

Clarity: Very slight inclusions

Origin

Discovered in India in the
17th century

Value

Estimated at $250 million

Residence

The Smithsonian Institution
Washington, D.C.

THE KOH-I-NOOR DIAMOND

Description

Carats: 105.6 carats

Cut: Oval brilliant cut

Color: Colorless

Clarity: Flawless

Origin

Discovered in India in the
13th century

Value

Estimated at $400 million

Residence

The crown of the
British Queen Mother

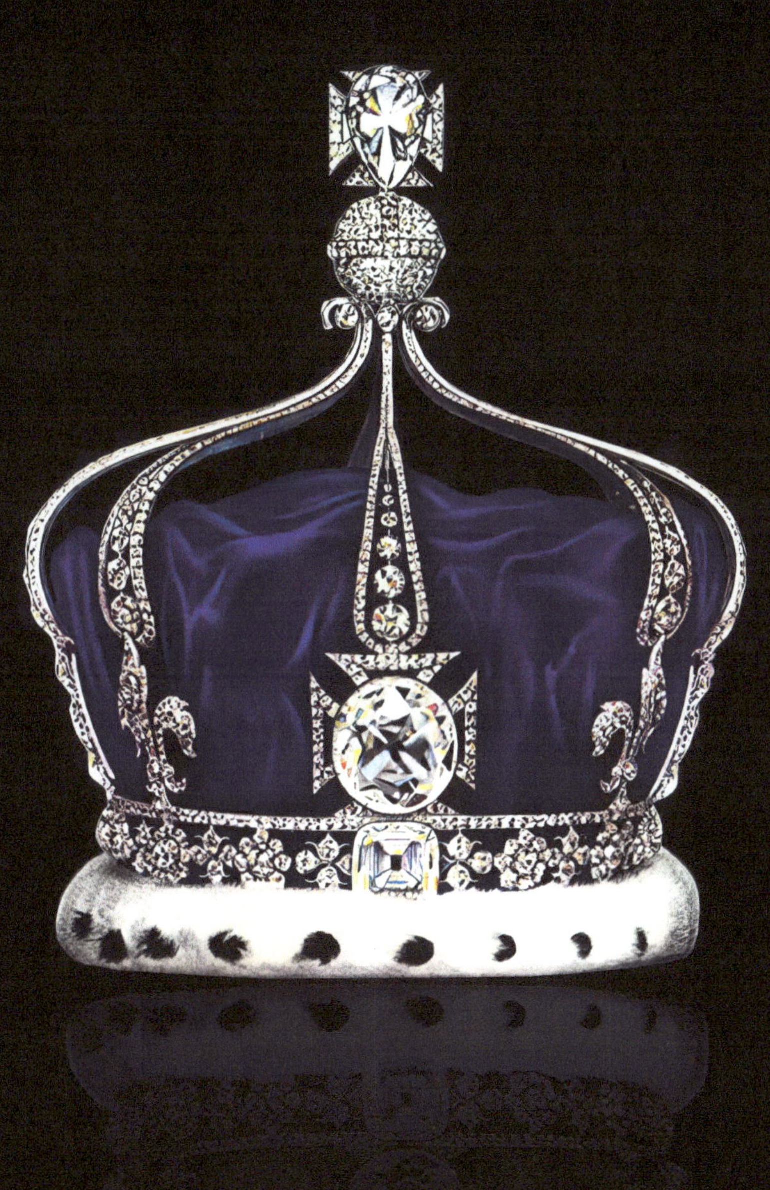

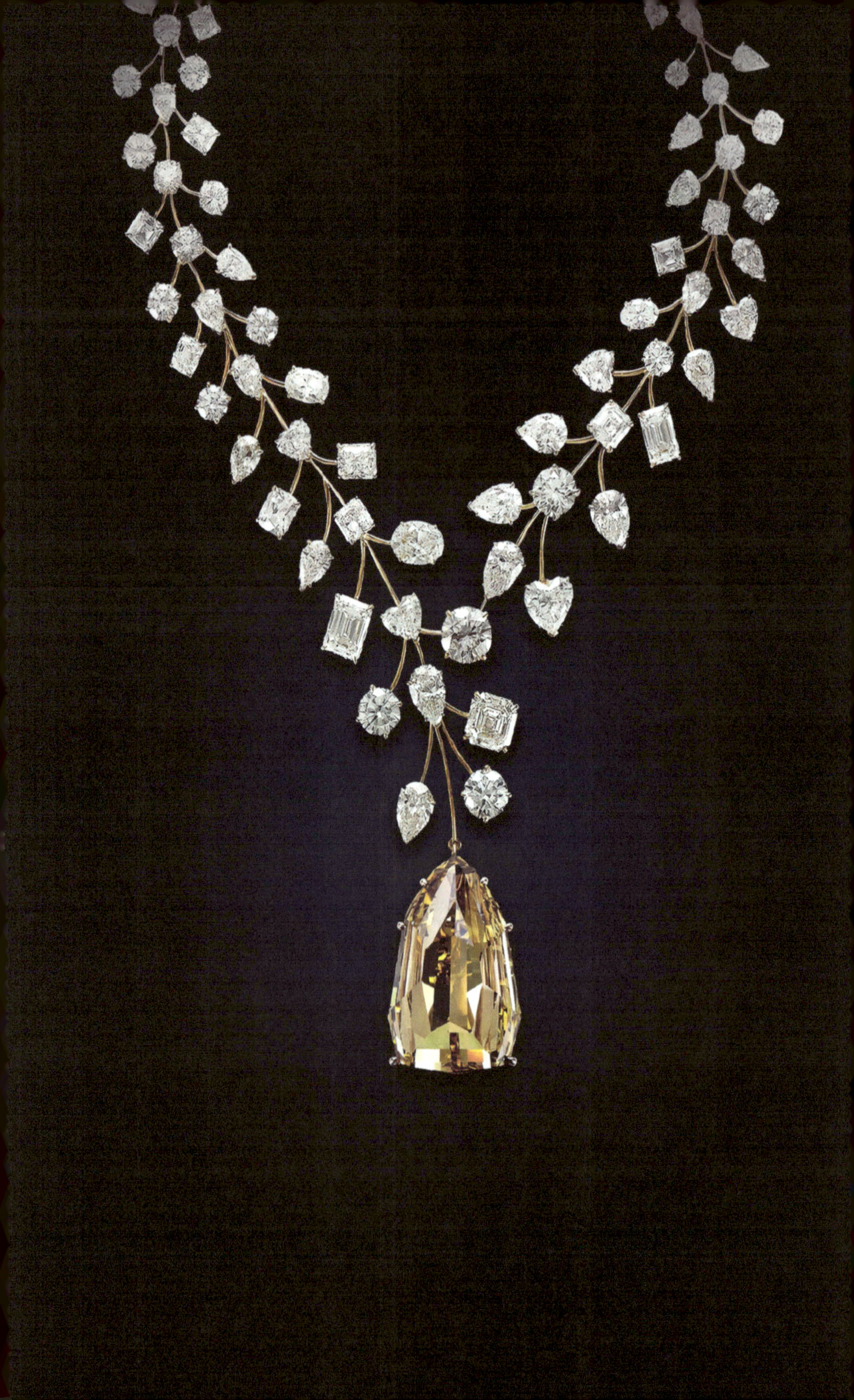

Description

Carats: 407.48 carats

Cut: Shield-shaped step cut

Color: Fancy brownish-yellow

Clarity: Flawless

Origin

Discovered in the African Congo
in the 1980s

Value

$55 million (entire necklace)

Residence

Owned by Mouawad, a luxury jeweler
based in Geneva, Switzerland

The Moussaieff Diamond

Description

Carats: 5.11 carats

Cut: Triangular brilliant cut

Color: Fancy red

Origin

Discovered by a Brazilian
farmer in 1989

Value

$20 million

Residence

Owned by Moussaieff Jewelers, Ltd.
London, England

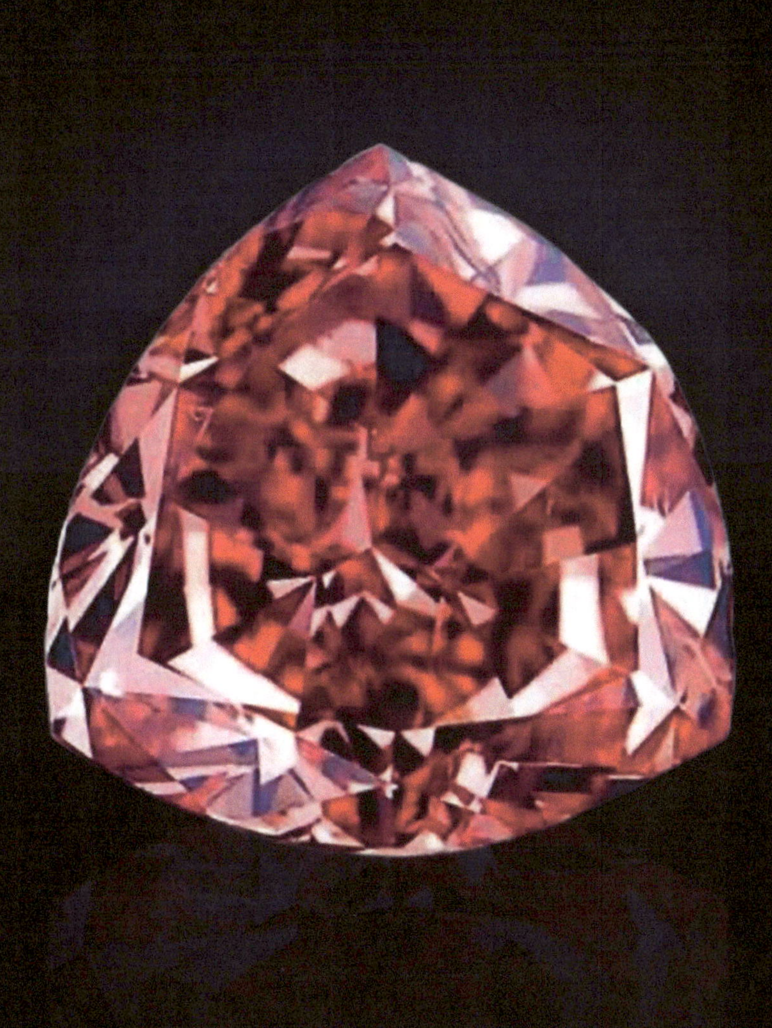

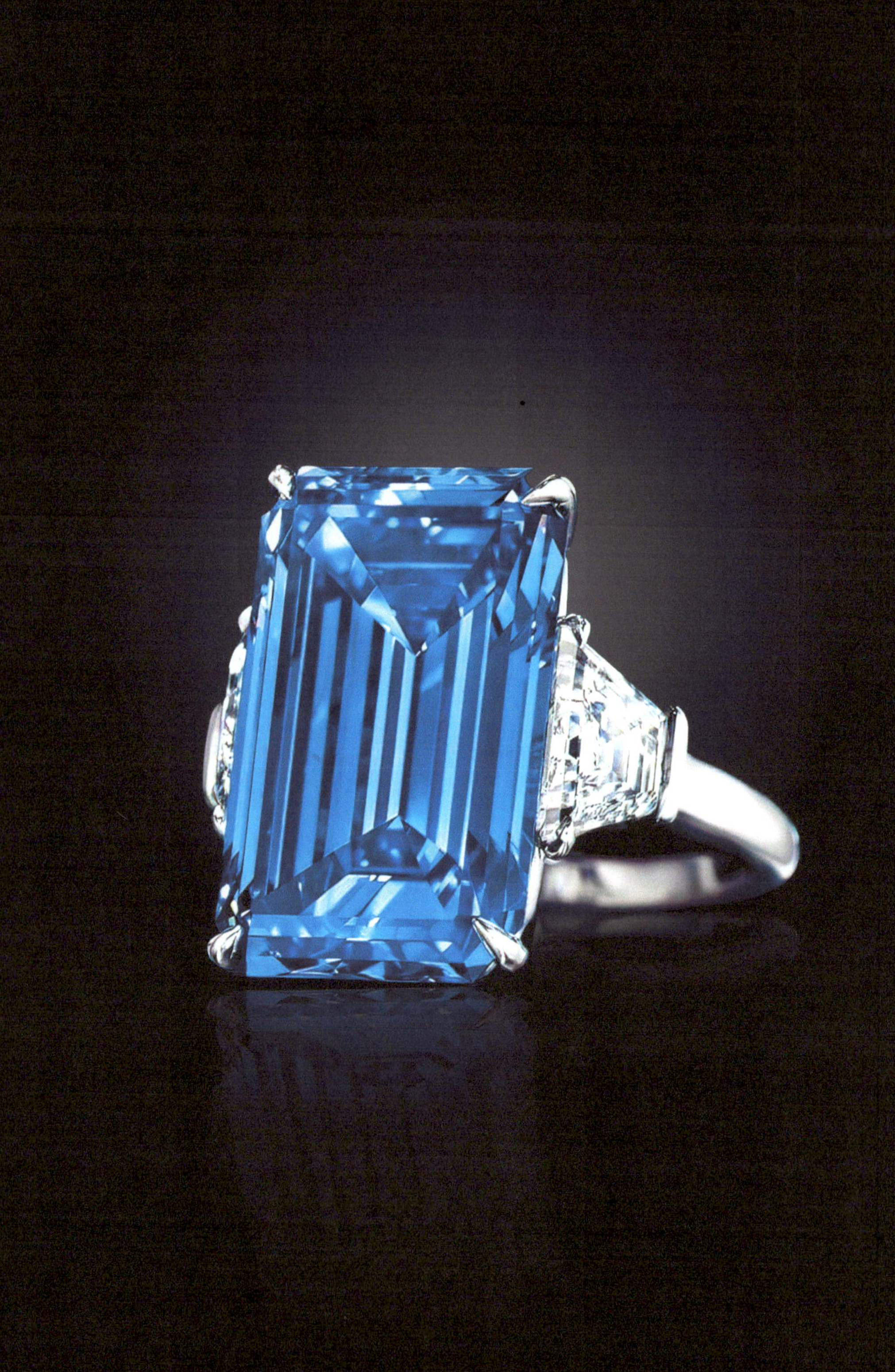

The Oppenheimer Blue

Description

Carats: 14.62 carats

Cut: Rectangular cut

Color: Vivid blue

Clarity: Very, very slightly included

Origin

Discovered in South Africa in the
early 20th century

Value

$57.5 million

Residence

Undisclosed

THE ORLOV

Description

Carats: 190 carats

Cut: Rose cut, half-egg shape

Color: Faint blue-green

Origin

Discovered in India in 1650

Value

Unknown

Residence

Mounted on the Russian
Imperial Sceptre on display at the
Kremlin Armory in Moscow

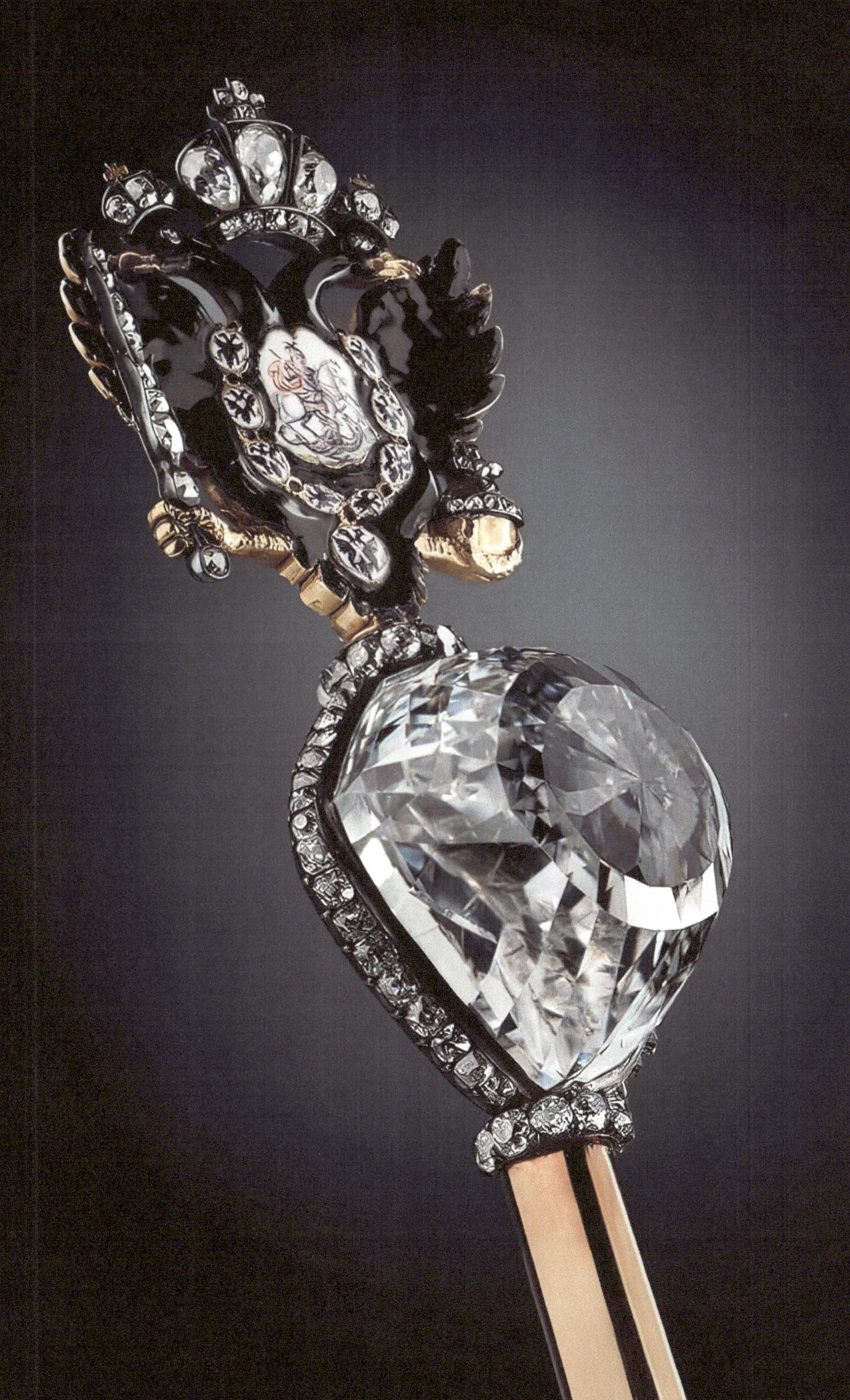

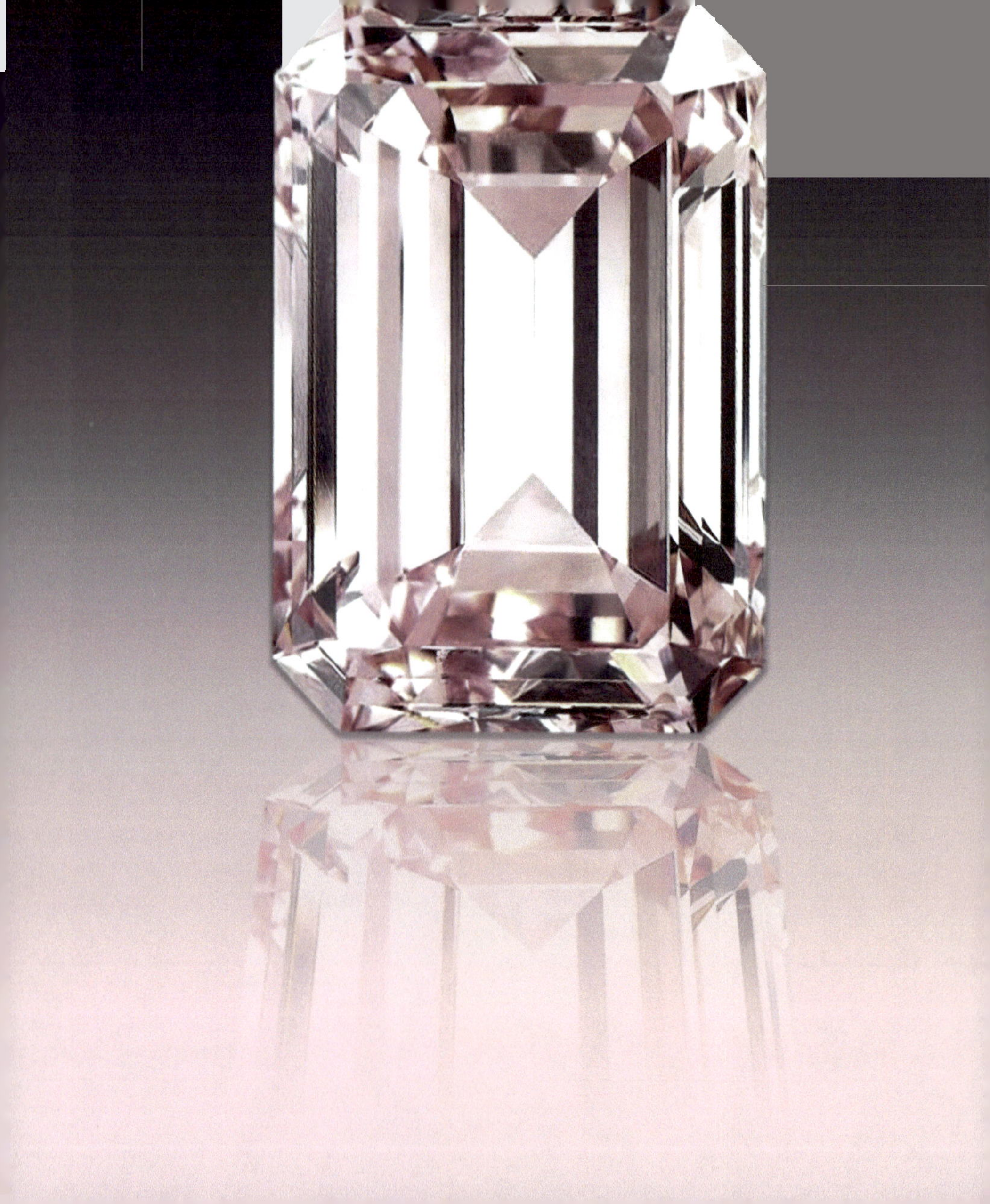

Description

Carats: 14.23 carats

Cut: Rectangular cut

Color: Fancy intense pink

Clarity: Very, very slight inclusions

Origin

Discovered in Australia

Value

$23.2 million

Residence

Undisclosed

THE PINK STAR

Description

Carats: 59.6 carats

Cut: Oval mixed cut

Color: Fancy vivid pink

Clarity: Flawless

Origin

Discovered in South Africa

in 1999

Value

$71.2 million

Residence

Owned by Hong Kong jeweler,

Chow Tai Fook

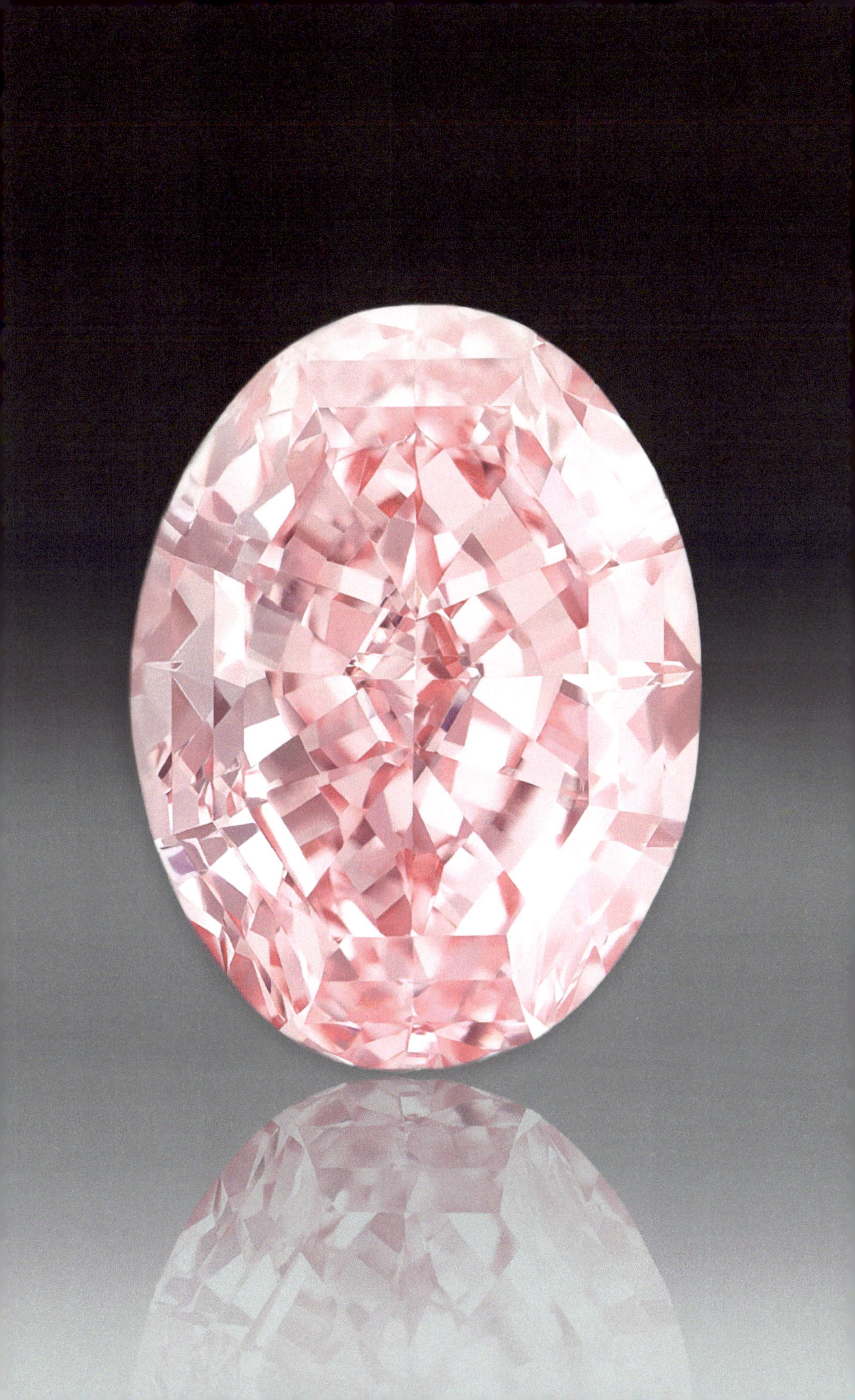

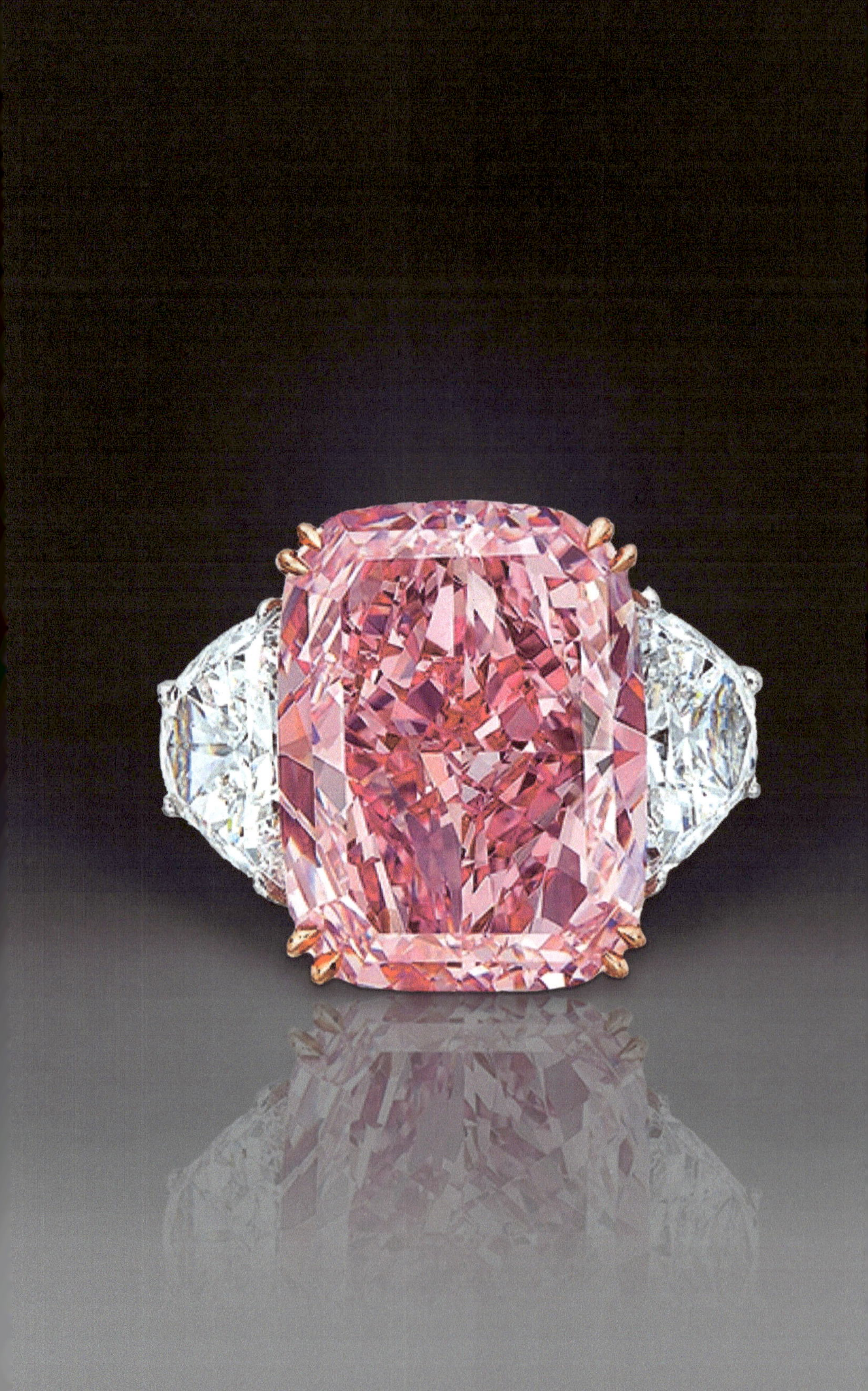

THE SAKURA

Description

Carats: 15.81 carats

Cut: Mixed cushion cut

Color: Fancy vivid purple-pink

Clarity: Flawless

Origin

Discovered in Russia

in 2017

Value

$29.3 million

Residence

Undisclosed

Description

Carats: 14.83 carats

Cut: Oval modified brilliant cut

Color: Fancy vivid purple-pink

Clarity: Flawless

Origin

Discovered in in Russia

in 2017

Value

$26.6 million

Residence

Undisclosed

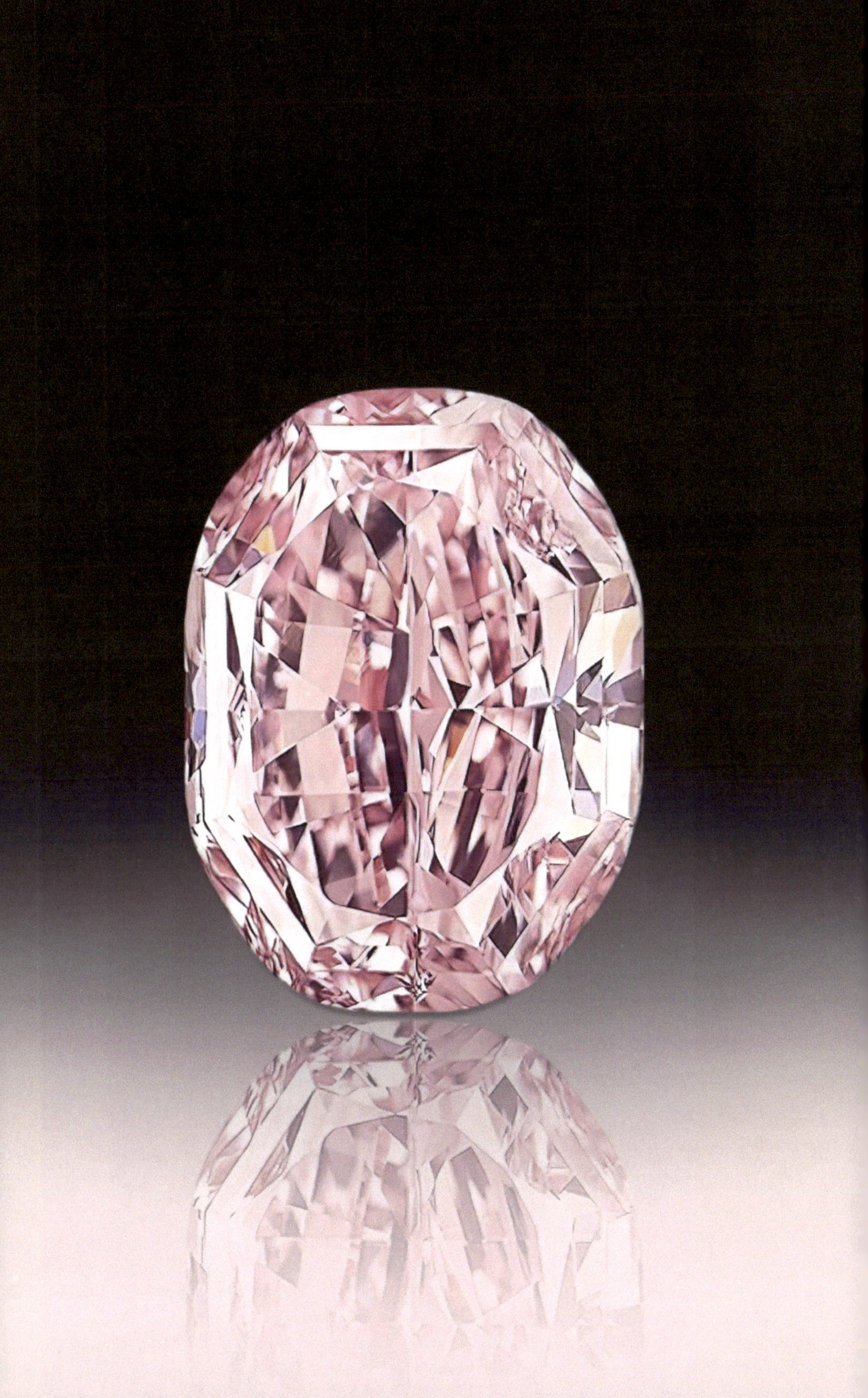

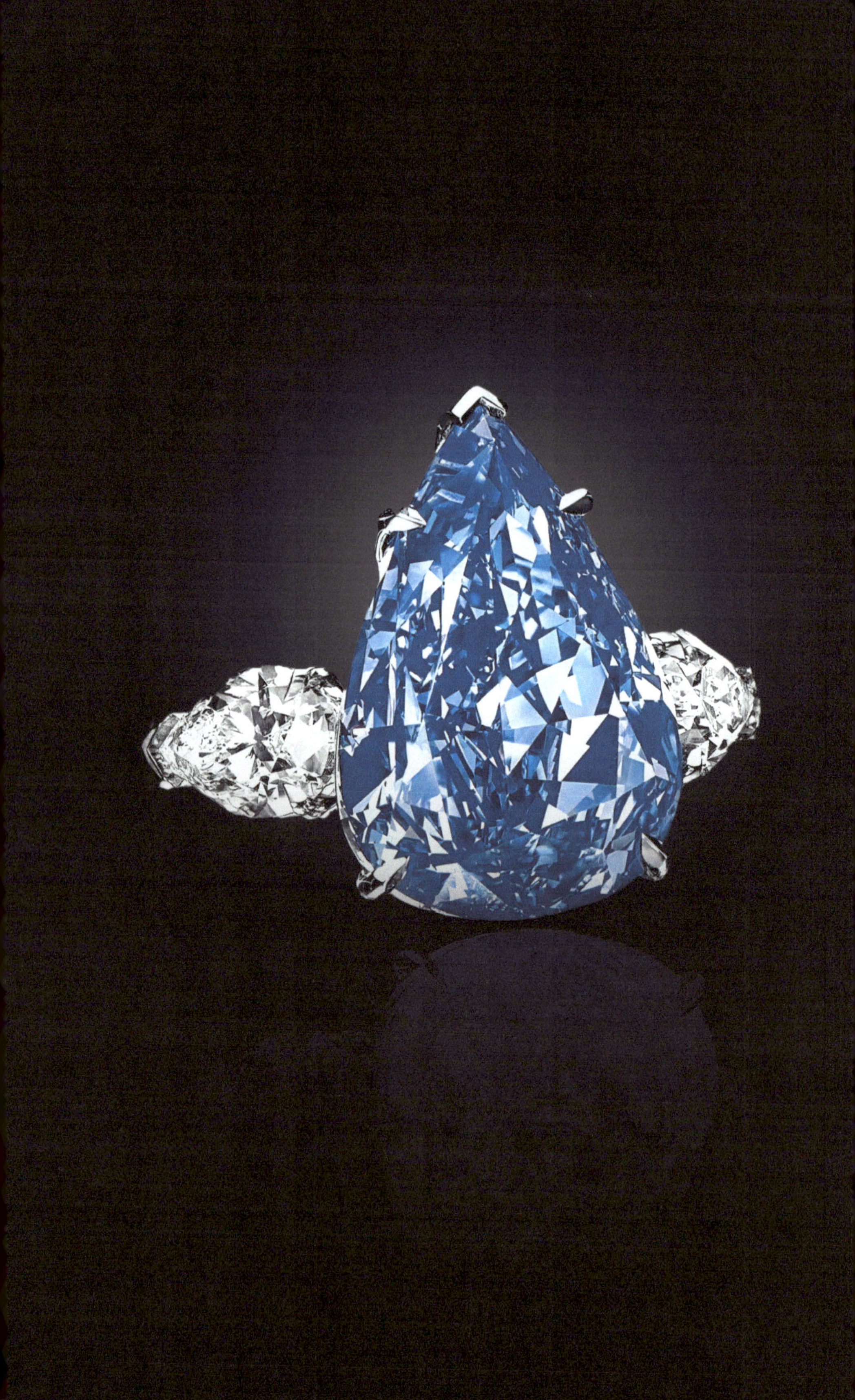

Description

Carats: 13.22 carats

Cut: Pear-shaped diamond cut

Color: Fancy vivid blue

Clarity: Flawless

Origin

Discovered in South Africa

Value

$23.8 million

Residence

Owned by luxury jewelry dealer,
Harry Winston, Inc.

Description

Carats: 31.06 carats

Cut: Antique oval stellar brilliant cut

Color: Fancy deep blue

Clarity: Flawless

Origin

Discovered in India in the
17th century

Value

$23.4 million

Residence

Owned by

Sheikh Hamad bin Khalifa Al Thani,
Father Emir of Qatar

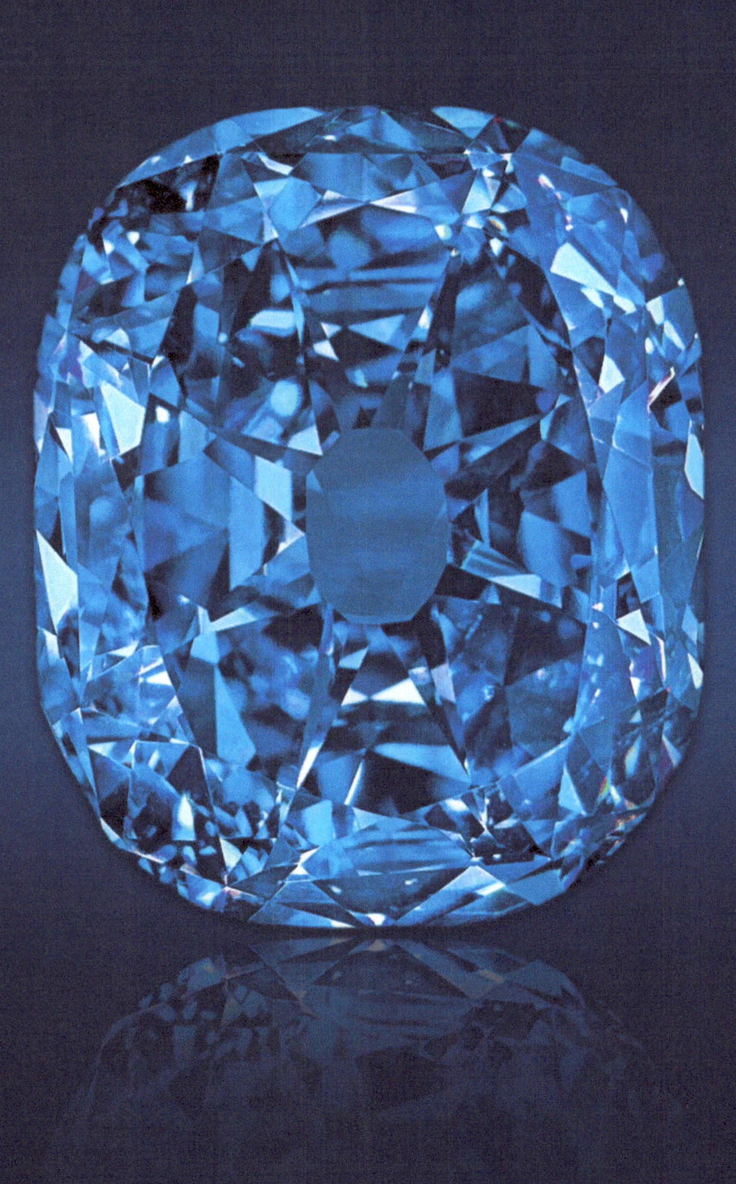